The Ultimate Vitamin B12 Deficiency Symptoms Book:

Causes and Treatment to fight and Regain your Life

Tom Will

Copyright © 2023 Tom Will

All rights reserved.

ISBN: 9798840825365

DEDICATION

I dedicate this book to myself.

CONTENTS

	Dedication	iii
1	Introduction	1
2	Symptoms of Vitamin B12 Deficiency - Understand How It Starts	4
3	Symptoms of Vitamin B12 Deficiency - Key Risk Groups	8
4	Benefits of Vitamin B12 (Methylcobalamin) Supplementation	12
5	Vitamin B12 Deficiency And Its Causes	17
6	Vitamin B12 Deficiency: Symptoms, Causes, Diagnosis, and Treatment	21
7	Vitamin B12 Absorption - How it Works and What Goes Wrong When it Doesn't	25
8	How to Take a B12 Supplement	28
9	Using Vitamin B-12 Tablets	31
10	Conclusion	37

INTRODUCTION

Many people who use vitamin B12 supplements are unaware that folate and vitamin B12 are part of the B complex and essential for healthy red blood cells. Vegetarians, especially vegans who don't consume dairy or meat, are especially in danger since vitamin B12 is seldom present in plants. To maintain appropriate levels of homocysteine in the blood, this vitamin B12 and folic acid are essential. So any shortage will result in various health issues.

Not because people are taking less vitamin B12 than is advised does a vitamin B12 deficit show symptoms. Every cell in the body is impacted by vitamin B12 deficiency, although the effects are most noticeable in the tissues where cells ordinarily cycle quickly, such as the gastrointestinal tract and the bone marrow, which produce blood. Additionally, a shortage may result in neurological abnormalities such as tingling and numbness in the hands and feet. Mood disorders, anxiety, restlessness, sleeplessness, and night terrors are all included. Additionally, it may cause weight gain, lethargy, nausea, constipation, weariness, weakness, and flatulence (gas). Similar to many other curable health issues, symptoms of vitamin B12 insufficiency might resemble those of Alzheimer's disease, senile dementia, and age-related dementia.

According to research by the Agricultural Research Service (ARS), osteoporosis may be related to the symptoms of B12 insufficiency, which also include poor balance, forgetfulness, and cognitive deterioration. Regardless of the underlying cause, severe vitamin B12 deficiency symptoms can include tongue burning, weakness, fatigue, loss of appetite, intermittent constipation and diarrhea, abdominal pain, weight loss, menstrual symptoms, psychological symptoms, and nervous system issues like tingling and numbness in the hands and feet. People with sub-clinical vitamin B12 deficiency may have sensory neuropathy, myelopathy, and encephalopathy within days or weeks after being exposed to nitrous oxide anesthesia.

We frequently overlook the vitamins and minerals that are so important to our physiological functioning because of fast-food attitude that so many of us adopt as a result of our fast-paced lives. You might be surprised by the negative impact that a daily lack of proper intake has on our body and mind. I want to focus on the signs and symptoms of vitamin B12 deficiency.

This supplement can have some extremely bad side effects on your body if you don't consume enough of it, including

- ✓ Tingling in the tongue: A solid indication that you might require vitamin D is if you experience tingling or itching around your mouth.
- ✓ Migraine attacks: Of course, there are numerous causes for these severe headaches, but one of them is a deficiency.

- ✓ Breathing difficulty: If you strain yourself and experience shortness of breath, it might be due to this ailment; however, if it is accompanied by chest pains, it could be due to heart disease.
- ✓ Mouth sores: Sores on the sides of your mouth are a clear indicator of Vitamin B12 deficiency and one of the basic symptoms.
- ✓ Facial spasm on one side: This is generally visible in the eye, but not always.
- ✓ Increased impatience and emotional sensitivity for things that did not affect you previously.

If you just have one symptom, it will not tell you if you have a deficit or not, but if you detect more than one symptom, you should see a doctor to receive a good treatment that will help you.

Chapter 1

SYMPTOMS OF VITAMIN B12 DEFICIENCY - UNDERSTAND HOW IT STARTS

The food we eat in a normal and healthy manner contains all of the nutrients we could ever need for a healthy lifestyle. Even so, maintaining a perfect balance of all nutrients in the body is not always possible. We always seem to be missing something. To compensate for these inadequacies, we must consume those nutrients in supplemental form. These are known as supplements. Any supplement use should be preceded by a consultation with a doctor. A lack of some nutrients may go virtually undetected, while a lack of others may have catastrophic consequences. As we all know, vitamin B12 is linked to the functioning of healthy nerve cells. It aids in the maintenance of red blood cell form and quantity. It also protects against heart disease and stroke. It also aids in the processing of DNA in our bodies. Any shortfall would cause the body to malfunction in these areas. Anemia is caused by a low amount of red blood cells. The person suffers from shortness of breath as a result of this (because of low oxygen supplied to the body). Basic vitamin B12 deficiency symptoms include dizziness, weariness, and poor energy. The gastrointestinal system and its functions are also affected by the deficit. It may also produce nausea, vomiting, gas, constipation, or diarrhea. All of these contribute to a loss of appetite and weight.

Since vitamin B12 aids in the healthy functioning of nerve cells, its lack has an impact on their health and function. If it is not recognized and treated promptly, it might cause lasting nerve cell damage. Numbness in the hands and feet, inability to balance, trouble walking, unusual depression, and memory loss are all symptoms.

The skin also exhibits indications of vitamin B12 insufficiency. Paleness of the cheeks and eyes, dryness of the lips, and other symptoms suggest a low blood count. In layman's terms, blood is the transporter of food and oxygen to all regions of the body. If the blood (in this example, low red blood cells) is harmed, the entire body and the functionality of all organs are destined to suffer. The more serious the shortage, the worse the repercussions. Though it may not be relevant in the beginning. It is critical to identify vitamin B12 deficiency symptoms early on so that they may be treated and supplements administered.

What signs might indicate a vitamin B12 deficiency?

The sooner you become aware of signs that might indicate a vitamin B12 shortage, the better. When the impacts are just mild to moderate, it is simple to write them off as aging because they can accumulate. There are various signs of vitamin B12 insufficiency, but some of the most prevalent ones are weakness, confusion, bleeding gums, irritability, agitation, lightheadedness, and constipation. Heart disease, stroke, and dementia like Alzheimer's disease can all have more severe long-term symptoms. Let's look at a couple of these vitamin B12 insufficiency symptoms.

Vitamin B12 is essential for the creation of red blood cells, hence a vitamin B12 deficit might result in fatigue. These blood cells assist in the efficient delivery of oxygen throughout our bodies. In addition to being essential for energy, a lack of red blood cells results in anemia. Anemia can make you feel weak and tired. Because this vitamin aids in proper food metabolization, a B-12 shortage can also contribute to sensations of exhaustion. A healthy metabolism of the food we eat aids in the conversion of carbs into glucose. When glucose is absorbed into your body, it provides you with energy.

Mood instability is another sign of a vitamin B-12 deficiency. Low amounts of this frequently disregarded vitamin can cause mood changes, anxiety, and depression. The brain chemical serotonin, which makes us feel happy, is produced in our brains with the aid of vitamin B12. Additionally, vitamin B12 aids in the production of melatonin, which controls our sleep patterns. Additionally, this vitamin helps to maintain the general function of our neurological system, which is crucial for optimal mental health.

Heart disease and artery hardening are two extremely dangerous B12 deficient symptoms. Homocysteine (HCY), a naturally occurring amino acid in our systems, has the potential to be hazardous if levels rise too high. HCY levels are kept under control with the use of vitamin B12. There can be serious damage at toxic amounts. This is due to the negative effects HCY has on the cells that make up our arteries and veins. Heart attacks and strokes may result from the injury.

There are Serious, Long-Term Effects of B-12 Deficiency
People who experience the effects of vitamin B12 insufficiency sometimes lament their inability to think properly or to recall details. These two symptoms are commonly disregarded and allowed to worsen because they

are incorrectly sometimes linked to "growing older." They may, regrettably, be a sign of dementia, which includes Alzheimer's disease. Dementia is characterized by a steady deterioration in cognitive ability. Dementia symptoms include memory loss, disorientation, a tendency to get lost easily, and paranoia. Sadly, dementia currently has no recognized treatment.

Even though these are not all the signs of a vitamin B12 shortage, they should help you understand how vital this mineral is for your wellbeing. Although there are many potential causes for these symptoms, it's still crucial to make sure you're taking enough B12 each day. Since B12 is regarded as non-toxic, it is practically impossible to consume too much of it. One of the best methods to avoid a major B12 deficit is to combine a nutritious diet with the use of a high-quality B12 supplement.

Chapter 2
SYMPTOMS OF VITAMIN B12 DEFICIENCY - KEY RISK GROUPS

Everyone can have vitamin B12 deficiency symptoms at some point in their lives for a variety of reasons (lack of appropriate nutrition, bad eating habits, etc.), but some people are more prone than others to be deficient. Knowing if you belong to one of these risk categories will help you raise your awareness and, ultimately, prevent a vitamin B12 deficit.

Vegetarians:

Vegetarians and vegans are deficient in B12 due to a lack of protein from animal-based meals. Vitamin B12 is found in meat, poultry, seafood, eggs, and dairy products. A diet lacking in these food sources lacks B12, to begin with, and they will rapidly become deficient in vitamin B12 unless nutritional supplements are given.

Vegetarian Diets for Pregnant and Lactating Women:

This group is more vulnerable than other vegetarians. During pregnancy and lactation, pregnant and lactating mothers require additional B12 for themselves and their babies. A typical adult needs 2.4 mcg per day, whereas pregnant women need 2.6 mcg per day and breastfeeding women need 2.8 mcg per day. Even pregnant women on low-meat diets should keep an eye out for vitamin B12 insufficiency symptoms to preserve their own and their babies' wellbeing. This group should take prenatal vitamins with a B12 supplement.

Adults aged 50 and up:

Atrophic gastritis affects around 30% of persons over the age of 50. This procedure affects the digestive tract and makes it more difficult for the body to absorb vitamin B12 in its normal condition (from natural foods). B12 nutritional supplements are synthetic and unaffected by atrophic gastritis, lowering the risk of vitamin B12 insufficiency.

Patients with Gastric Bypass and Gastrointestinal Disease:

Surgery, Chron's disease, celiac disease, and ulcerative colitis all disrupt the normal digestive process, making it extremely difficult for the body to absorb vitamin B12. I'll publish a separate essay about the specifics of these conditions, but nutritional supplements should be examined (preferably in a non-swallowed form). This population is at significant risk of vitamin B12 deficiency.

Common Reasons for Vitamin B12 Deficiency

There are several causes of vitamin B12 insufficiency that one may experience. Some folks don't have the necessary inherent component to digest this chemical adequately. This often manifests early in life but can also happen as you get older; unfortunately, it is frequently misdiagnosed.

Vegans may also lack some nutrients since their diet

prevents them from consuming sources of food that come from animals. Unfortunately, animal sources are the only places to get vitamin B12. B12 pills will guarantee that there are no problems.

Elderly persons should also take tablets that include vitamin B12. 15 percent of persons over 65 have vitamin B12 deficiencies, according to research. A decrease in the gastrointestinal system, which leads to inadequate nutrition absorption, is a contributing factor in this. Sublingual or injectable versions of B12 are the ideal delivery methods for the elderly since they skip the digestive processes.

The use of stomach acid-blocking devices and medications, which can lower vitamin B12 levels, is another cause of B12 insufficiency. People with illnesses that cause malabsorption, such as Celiac disease, low stomach acid, or those who have undergone stomach or intestinal surgery, are also affected by this. Poor nutrition absorption may be caused by any gastric issue.

An extremely safe and cost-effective dietary supplement, vitamin B12 has several advantages. Proper supplementation might be crucial for everyone who is worried about their health.

Try taking a coenzyme form of B12, often methylcobalamin, plus a B-Complex vitamin with folic acid for two weeks if you have any of the signs or problems linked to a vitamin B12 deficiency.

If you experience any advantages, that are terrific; if not, there's no damage done. If your symptoms persist, you should always consult a doctor. One intriguing idea concerning vitamin B12 is that in the second century, the Romans recorded oysters as an aphrodisiac meal. Could it be that many Romans were B12 deficient, and that eating oysters—which are high in B12—cured them of their deficiencies, restoring their youthfulness and vigor? It is possible.

Chapter 3
BENEFITS OF VITAMIN B12 (METHYLCOBALAMIN) SUPPLEMENTATION

Vitamin B12 is one of the most underrated dietary supplements available. In addition to other B vitamins, your body requires this vitamin to produce healthy DNA, keep your energy levels stable, and maintain a healthy neurological system. These are all crucial processes for your daily life.

Feeling exhausted and sluggish is the main sign of a vitamin B12 deficiency. The B-complex vitamins are crucial for the breakdown of carbohydrates and the creation of energy. This system can malfunction and result in these symptoms if it is missing all of the necessary parts. B12 deficiency can cause Pernicious Anemia, a dangerous medical illness, if it is not diagnosed or treated. Shortness of breath, weariness, fast heartbeat, lack of appetite, diarrhea, tingling and numbness in the hands and feet, painful mouth, unsteady stride, especially in the dark, issues with the tongue, poor sense of smell, and bleeding gums are all signs of a B12 deficiency. A high folic acid consumption might mask a B12 deficiency. By include B12-rich foods in your diet or by taking supplements, this problem is readily treated. The majority of the time, a B-Complex vitamin and a folic acid supplement should be given together with vitamin B12.

There has been a marked rise in vitamin B12 insufficiency as a result of altered diets and highly processed food. Fish, dairy products, eggs, and red meat all contain vitamin B12. Vegetables are not known sources of vitamin B12. Organ meat consumption was formerly extremely prevalent, but today it's rare to see steak and kidney pie or liver and onions in a fast food joint. Diets that are nutritionally balanced have decreased as a result of contemporary diets. Mollusks/clams (85 micrograms per 3 ounce piece) and cow liver are the best sources of B12 (47 micrograms per 3oz portion). The degradation of vitamins might occur as a result of overcooking.

If you don't like oysters or organ meat, vitamin B12 pills will work just well. This guide will assist you in selecting the best B12 supplement for your requirements as there are several different types of the vitamin. If unsure, speak with your doctor or take methylcobalamin.

A physiologically active coenzyme form of vitamin B12 is methylcobalamin. This indicates that it is already in a form that your body can utilize and does not need to undergo any metabolic modifications. Due to the molecule's modification by your digestive system, the medicine is available as a sublingual pill that dissolves beneath your tongue. The vitamin can quickly help you thanks to the sublingual method's immediate bloodstream entry.

Cyanocobalamin is a synthetic, inactive version of vitamin B12 that has to undergo many metabolic steps in order to be useful. When someone has specific deficits or health problems, this might be troublesome. Sadly, this is the most widely available form of vitamin B12 on the market and is present in the majority of vitamin B-Complexes.

The non-active form of vitamin B12 known as hydroxycobalamin is frequently administered intravenously. Depending on your condition, it provides a variety of advantages. For people who are sensitive to cyanide, it is advised. By interacting with the molecule to create cyanocobalamin, which can subsequently be eliminated from the body, hydroxycobalamin aids in the body's ability to bind free cyanide. Although cyanide is widely known to be extremely harmful, the body constantly employs it in very tiny amounts for metabolic functions.

The other coenzyme form of vitamin B12 that is physiologically active is adenosylcobalamin. Typically, this type is sold as an injectable and is only accessible with a prescription.

Benefits of Vitamin B12

A safe, reliable, and reasonably priced vitamin is vitamin B12. A regular consumption of a certain amount of vitamin B12 is crucial for maintaining a balance in the body for health-conscious people. B12 can be consumed orally or intravenously as supplements. It can also be derived through dietary sources.

When combined with other B-group vitamins, vitamin B12 guarantees the efficient operation of the body's essential biological functions. It is crucial for producing DNA and preserving a healthy neurological system. Red blood cell production in the body is regulated by vitamin B12. The significance that vitamin B12 plays in sustaining and boosting the body's energy levels is only one of its many advantages.

The benefits of vitamin B12 come in many different forms.

The coenzyme form of vitamin B12, methylcobalamin, is a body-friendly form since there are no metabolic processes necessary for its absorption, and it may be utilised in its natural state. A sublingual pill that dissolves beneath the tongue is available (because the digestive system might modify this molecule). This process allows vitamin B12 to enter the circulation immediately, which has a number of advantages. Another vitamin B12 form known as hydroxycobalamin has been proven to be successful in treating cyanide poisoning.

A clear negative relationship between homocysteine (an amino acid present in the human body) levels and vitamin B12 levels has been demonstrated by research. Homocysteine production inhibition causes endothelial dysfunction, which results in artery constriction and is a precursor to atherosclerosis; vitamin B12 works to prevent atherosclerosis. A vitamin B12 supplement improves the effectiveness of folic acid's ability to reduce homocysteine levels. According to research, an appropriate intake of vitamin B12 works in concert with folic acid to prevent thrombosis and heart disease. The combination of folate and vitamin B12 is necessary for the production of S-adenosylmethionine (SAMe), a substance implicated in immune system and mood function.

Others That May Be At Risk Of B12 Deficiency

Pernicious anemia sufferers may be more vulnerable. When red blood cells don't contain enough hemoglobin to transport oxygen to the cells and tissues, anemia develops. Fatigue and weakness are typical signs. Numerous health issues, such as a lack of iron, vitamin B12, vitamin B6, and vitamin B6 can arise from anemia. More than a century ago, a deadly B12 shortage brought on by stomach atrophy was known as pernicious anemia. Due to this disease, the stomach cells are unable to secrete intrinsic factor. To be absorbed by the system, B12 has to bind with IF. When a person has this illness, they are typically given a B12 injection to raise their levels to the appropriate levels, and then supplements to keep them there. This therapy must be overseen by a primary care physician.

Due to impaired absorption, people with gastrointestinal issues may be low in B12. Cohn's disease, celiac disease, and individuals who have had gastrointestinal surgery, such as the removal of all or part of the stomach, may be some of these illnesses. Cells that are in charge of manufacturing intrinsic factor may die as a result of this.

Atrophic gastritis, which is an increased proliferation of intestinal bacteria, may affect up to 30% of adults over 50. Gastric juice production is reduced as a result of this, and the extra bacteria may actually compete with one another for the limited B12 supply. They are unable to typically absorb vitamin B12 as a result. However, they may absorb synthetic B12, such as that found in nutritional supplements and fortified meals. The finest B12 sources for adults over 50 may come from these two sources.

Vegans and strict vegetarians run the danger of acquiring B12 deficiency. This is because they do not ingest animal products, which are where B12 is derived from. Cereals with added B12 are an excellent source for this population.

Chapter 4
VITAMIN B12 DEFICIENCY AND ITS CAUSES

Let talk more about the reasons of a vitamin B12 shortage in this post. Let's first examine the roles that vitamin B12 plays in the body. The so-called vitamin B complex, which includes vitamin B12, is essential for preserving the healthy operation of the brain and nerves. Additionally, it is highly helpful in the creation of DNA molecules and the recovery of the body's damaged cells. It encourages our bodies to cleanse from different harmful substances.

What Leads to a Deficiency in Vitamin B12?
Aging and a lack of vitamin B12 in the diet are the two main causes of vitamin B12 insufficiency. There are, of course, some other factors, mostly medical ones. These are what they are:

One of the most frequent medical reasons for a vitamin B12 deficiency is pernicious anemia. It might be thought of as a particular sort of anemia, mostly brought on by the intestines' inability to absorb vitamin B12. When the intrinsic factor cannot be produced by the stomach mucosa, this occurs. It might be characterized as a glycoprotein that is essential for absorbing vitamin B12.

A serious problem with vitamin B12 insufficiency affects

vegetarians as well. This occurs as a result of their preference for vegetables over meat, which is a poor source of vitamin B12 and which they avoid consuming. Since it is commonly recognized that plants do not make good supplies of this vitamin, a diet consisting solely of plants is likely to leave one deficient in it.

The Crohn's Disease is a further medical factor that merits notice. It really causes gut inflammation, which can cause a number of unpleasant symptoms. At the same time, vitamin B12 absorption is hindered. Whenever we discuss gastrointestinal issues, we must bring up Diphyllobothrium Latum. It is a syndrome that develops when raw seafood, such as sushi, is ingested often.

Another gastrointestinal condition that results in the loss of stomach glandular cells is atrophic gastroenteritis. This causes damage to pepsin and intrinsic factor, which results in megaloblastic anemia and vitamin insufficiency.

A lack of vitamin B12 might result from taking certain drugs. Fortunately, a healthy diet that includes foods high in vitamin B12 can quickly and effectively treat a vitamin B12 shortage. It is usually sufficient to consume animal items like meat, eggs, milk, and dairy goods. The use of vitamin B12 supplements is advised for vegetarians, but only after consulting with a physician.

Is Sublingual Vitamin B12 Good For You? Get The Facts
There is a lot of information available on vitamin supplements, most of it contradictory, and there is no guidance as to where to go for the true facts about the vitamin supplements you might be thinking about taking. When a doctor advises you to take a specific vitamin

supplement, you'll frequently rush to the pharmacy without thinking twice and follow their instructions, frequently without knowing what the supplement is. Nevertheless, you should always be aware of the advantages of any supplement you might be instructed to take, as well as any potential adverse effects. You should be aware of the health advantages of starting the sublingual vitamin b12 if you have been advised to do so or just opted to do so for personal reasons.

Sublingual vitamin B12 is instantly absorbed into your circulation, making it useful as soon as you take it. When ingesting sublingual b12, you just place the tablet beneath your tongue and wait for it to dissolve rather than eating it with a glass of water. By doing this, the vitamin is rapidly absorbed as opposed to having to go through the lengthy digestive process. Your body will start to experience the effects of taking this vitamin as soon as it is absorbed into your bloodstream. You'll get healthier and more active as a result of this.

The following advantages are provided by sublingual vitamin B12:

- Improved Memory
- Enhanced Energy
- Better Mood
- Increased Focus
- Battles Sickness

Together, all of these advantages contribute to a healthy, whole individual. You are less likely to be late or forgetful if you have a strong memory. This will enhance both your personal and professional lives by making people perceive you as trustworthy and responsible. More energy allows you to play with and take care of your children, if you have any, as well as complete more of your goals. We all prefer happiness over sadness. Positivity can enable you to overcome any obstacles that may arise during your life. You can achieve the objectives you set for yourself if you maintain concentration. Of course, preventing sickness may be seen as the key advantage of taking this vitamin. When you regularly take this vitamin supplement, you'll live longer and be happier.

B12 supplementation will boost and improve many aspects of your life. This vitamin can help you fulfill your demands and maintain a positive and focused perspective on anything may come your way because life is so hectic these days for almost everyone. You may become physically and mentally fit by following a regular vitamin consumption plan. By establishing this as a practice today, you can subsequently ensure that you fully enjoy the advantages of regular vitamin consumption.

Chapter 5
VITAMIN B12 DEFICIENCY: SYMPTOMS, CAUSES, DIAGNOSIS, AND TREATMENT

Vitamin B12 is naturally present in animal foods such as meat, fish, eggs, and dairy products.

Vitamin B12 is an essential component that aids in the health of the body's nerves and blood cells. A lack of vitamin B12 can result in a variety of symptoms, including fatigue, weakness, constipation, loss of appetite, weight loss, and megaloblastic anemia. A vitamin B12 shortage, if left untreated, can lead to major health complications such as neurological disorders and pernicious anemia. The best strategy to avoid vitamin B12 shortage is to consume a well-balanced diet that contains vitamin B12-rich foods such as meat, fish, poultry, eggs, and dairy products.

Vitamin B12 shortage can result in a variety of symptoms and health issues. If you feel you are low in vitamin B12, you should consult a doctor for a diagnosis and therapy. Fatigue, weakness, feeling lightheaded or dizzy, pale complexion, headache, upset stomach, constipation, or diarrhea are all symptoms of vitamin B12 insufficiency. Tingling or numbness in your hands and feet is also possible. Vitamin B12 insufficiency can cause visual loss and cognitive issues in extreme situations.

Vitamin B12 is naturally present in animal foods such as meat, fish, eggs, and dairy products. A lack of vitamin B12 can result in a variety of symptoms, including fatigue, weakness, constipation, loss of appetite, and weight loss. Vitamin B12 deficiency can cause developmental delays in children. Anemia and neuropathy can also be caused by a lack of vitamin B12 (nerve damage).

Pernicious anemia, a form of autoimmune illness that destroys the stomach lining and hinders the body from correctly absorbing vitamin B12, is the most prevalent cause of vitamin B12 deficiency. Celiac disease, Crohn's disease, stomach surgery, and some drugs are also causes of vitamin B12 insufficiency (such as metformin). Vitamin B12 deficiency can result in a variety of symptoms, some of which are life-threatening. Symptoms might appear gradually over months or even years, or they can appear abruptly and be severe. Fatigue is the most prevalent symptom of vitamin B12 insufficiency. You may be always fatigued and lack the energy to accomplish things you typically love. Other early symptoms include sadness, memory issues, mood changes, and headaches.

Do you frequently feel tired and exhausted? Do you struggle with concentration or memory? These symptoms might indicate a vitamin B12 shortage. Vitamin B12 is a vitamin found in red meat, fowl, fish, and milk. It aids in the production of red blood cells and the appropriate functioning of the neurological system. Anemia and neurological disorders can result from a lack of vitamin B12. Consult your doctor if you believe you may be deficient in vitamin B12. He or she may request a blood test to determine your vitamin B12 levels.

Vitamin B12 deficiency can cause a variety of symptoms,

including fatigue, depression, impaired memory, and eyesight and balance issues. The most prevalent cause of vitamin B12 shortage is pernicious anemia, a disorder that interferes with the body's capacity to absorb this essential mineral. Vitamin B12 deficiency is often treated by taking supplements or receiving frequent injections of the vitamin.

Vitamin B12 is a necessary component that aids in the health of the body's nerves and blood cells. It also helps to produce DNA, RNA, and red blood cells. discolored in a certain way Vitamin B12 is often present in animal-derived foods such as meat, poultry, eggs, and dairy products. You may develop a deficit if you do not consume enough of these foods or if your body does not absorb Vitamin B12 effectively. Anemia - exhaustion, weakness, shortness of breath, and heart palpitations caused by a shortage of red blood cells - is the most prevalent sign of Vitamin B12 insufficiency. If left untreated, Vitamin B12 deficiency can cause a variety of health issues, including memory loss and dementia.

Vitamin B12 is an essential ingredient that the body needs for various key processes. Unfortunately, vitamin B12 insufficiency is rather widespread, affecting one out of every four persons. Vitamin B12 insufficiency symptoms might be modest and appear gradually. Fatigue, weakness, lightheadedness, fast pulse, headaches, memory issues, and trouble pronouncing words are some of the symptoms (making them sound muddled). More serious symptoms, such as tingling in the extremities (arms and legs), visual issues, and paranoia, might develop over time. Vitamin B12 deficiency can cause severe brain damage if left untreated.

Should I Supplement Vitamin B12?
Most people who routinely consume animal products don't require vitamin B12 supplements. A medical expert should

be consulted for therapy if the individual has a condition that restricts or prevents normal B12 absorption.

If vegetarians consume enough fish, milk, eggs, and other animal products, they may not need to take supplements. But it's crucial to remember that milk only has 0.45 g per 100 grams and eggs only have 0.89 g per 100 grams (eggs also have a property that slightly inhibits B12 absorption).

Vegans are most at risk for B12 insufficiency since they are prohibited from consuming any animal products, which are the sole sources of vitamin B12 in diet (except for artificially fortified foods). It's crucial for devout vegans to consume enough fortified foods or take vitamin B12 supplements to achieve or surpass the RDA.

In conclusion, there doesn't appear to be an Upper Limit (UL), assuming oral intake, hence supplementing with vitamin B12 is unlikely to have any adverse effects. For those who regularly consume animal products, supplements are typically not essential, although proponents contend that consuming B12 at levels considerably over the RDA has additional advantages. Although there seems to be a wide range of safe amounts of intake, the data addressing the optimal levels of vitamin B12 consumption is still unclear.

Chapter 6
VITAMIN B12 ABSORPTION - HOW IT WORKS AND WHAT GOES WRONG WHEN IT DOESN'T

The body's cells utilize cyanocobalamin, or vitamin B12, to process energy, and it is vitally necessary for life. This vitamin, which is mostly found in animal products, is absorbed through a complex and sensitive process that involves several crucial organs in the body. Even one of these signs going wrong might result in a serious B12 deficiency and a host of related ailments. In this post, we'll examine the steps involved in vitamin B12 absorption in the digestive tract, potential pitfalls, and the best B12 supplementation forms.

Without a perfectly calibrated mechanism, the body finds it relatively challenging to absorb B12, which is found in dairy and meat. First, the vitamin is "ridden" into the stomach by saliva molecules. After being digested by stomach acid and pancreatic enzymes, it binds to an "intrinsic factor" molecule in the stomach. In the small intestine, the B12 and intrinsic factor mixture can then be absorbed.

You got everything, right? Small intestines, stomach acid, pancreatic enzymes, and intrinsic factors. The appropriate operation of each of these four systems is necessary for vitamin B12 absorption. What are a few instances of potential problems? The stomach cells that generate intrinsic factors are unexpectedly attacked by the body due to a condition termed "pernicious anemia." Absence of intrinsic factor and B12. Sometimes IBS can lead to a plugged gut, which causes poor absorption in the small intestine. No small intestine, no B12. What occurs then if B12 is not well absorbed?

This causes anemia, which, if unchecked, might potentially cause brain damage. Although any B12 deficiency symptoms are sometimes referred to as "pernicious anemia," the phrase technically only describes the aforementioned inflammatory illness that causes B12 deficiency. However, the only way to treat the anemia is with a B12 pill.

B12 is a vitamin that may be bought and used orally for general usage. This is typically insufficient for someone who is unable to absorb it adequately since a pill will merely pass through the digestive system and encounter the same issues. However, B12 injections entirely avoid the digestive system and deliver the vitamin directly into circulation. The "sublingual" B12 tablet, which has been proved to be almost as effective as the injections are given a big enough dosage, may still occasionally be prescribed by a doctor.

Without vitamin B12, the body simply cannot operate, and insufficient absorption can cause nerve damage and deadly anemia. The absorption process is so intricate that a variety of issues might arise at any one of its many stages, and several disorders could disrupt this system. Your doctor would likely recommend B12 injectable supplementation if you have poor B12 absorption since oral pills just don't work well enough. However, if you are only taking B12 as a preventative measure, you should think about taking a B complex rather than just B12, as all the B vitamins act in harmony, and a deficit in one might result in imbalances that can be problematic.

Why Diabetics Should Check Their Vitamin B12 Levels Regularly

A well-known water-soluble vitamin called vitamin B12 is required for a variety of metabolic processes as well as the avoidance of several medical issues, most often hematological illnesses and spinal cord-related neuropathies (additional details on these disorders will be summarized in future publications). Cobalamin and cyanocobalamin are other names for vitamin B12 (the form found in most over-the-counter supplements). Cobalamin is the term given to it because it includes cobalt, which is part of the reason for its chemical structure. Humans are unable to manufacture or generate vitamins on their own, thus we must get them from food sources, bacteria found in our natural flora, and/or supplementation. Vitamins are, therefore "essential to life."

Chapter 7
HOW TO TAKE A B12 SUPPLEMENT

Do you eat only raw or vegan foods?

If so, you should be very careful with vitamin B12. Given that it is mostly generated in the intestines of animals, vitamin B12 is exceedingly difficult to get if one does not consume animal products (including ourselves). But unless you're getting B12 from other animals, you really need to supplement with a high quality B12 vitamin since our own B12 that we made is not absorbed effectively enough to maintain us up to the levels needed for optimal health.

One interesting aspect of this knowledge is that we could obtain B12 from plant meals hundreds of years ago when our food was cultivated in the healthiest soil with well-nourished animal fertilizer. But today, it is very hard to obtain enough B12 from conventional food stores or even organic farms. We must thus seek for alternative sources.

For the first several years on a vegan diet, you'll be OK because our bodies have a 3-year supply of vitamin B12. To be cautious, you should think about taking a tiny B12 supplement sometimes or seeing the doctor every year to have your blood levels of homocysteine and B vitamins checked.

Do not let more than three years pass without addressing this problem. When your body's B12 reserves are depleted, you may start to experience headaches, memory loss, skin problems, exhaustion, and digestive and skin-related problems.

Positively, B12 is excellent for energy, mood, and heart health. Consequently, everyone wins.

Best Foods for B12? Clams, oysters, liver, caviar, octopus, fish, crab, beef, lamb, cheese, and eggs are among more delicacies. Therefore, get out your money and treat yourself to some B12 if you do consume animal products. Or, in the sake of your health, request that someone else treat you to a fine supper.

There are various vegan B12 sources. B12 is typically added during manufacture of nutritional yeast, kombucha, and certain sea algae. However, even these aren't a sufficient or reliable supply, so you must decide whether to take a vitamin supplement or receive your B12 from animal sources.

When trying to find a reliable B12 dietary supplement. Choose one that has had little processing and no preservatives. Additionally, a liquid B12 in dropper form is the finest option. Typically, one dropper contains more than you require for one day. Take it and hold the liquid for 30 seconds beneath your tongue. The easiest way to absorb vitamins into the bloodstream and start working is by placing them beneath the tongue.

Vitamin B12 Deficiency - What You Don't Know CAN Hurt You!

Eating a meal that contains all the nourishment that our bodies need is one of the toughest things to achieve in today's fast-paced environment. So much of the food we eat is either heavily processed or it was cultivated in nutrient-poor soil. Because of this, many of our foods are deficient in vitamins and minerals. We try our best to eat healthfully and believe that taking a multivitamin will make up for any deficiencies in our diet. Unfortunately, despite our best efforts, we frequently fall well short of providing our bodies with what they require. Thus, over time, we may become critically deficient in important vitamins and minerals.

A typical insufficiency is vitamin B12 deficiency. At least four out of ten Americans suffer from a clinical B12 deficiency. Millions of individuals only consume this essential vitamin in sufficient amounts to get by. Unbeknownst to most individuals, vitamin B12 insufficiency happens far more commonly. Many people have daily vitamin B12 insufficiency symptoms without even being aware of it. From minor to to significant, vitamin B12 insufficiency symptoms might present. The long-term effects of a B12 deficiency can be fatal if it persists for many years.

Chapter 8
USING VITAMIN B-12 TABLETS

Follow all instructions on the product packaging before taking the over-the-counter drug if you're using it for self-treatment. Ask your pharmacist any queries you may have. Follow your doctor's instructions if you have been told to take this medicine.

Take this medicine by mouth as prescribed by your doctor or the product label, generally once day with or without meal. To get the most out of this product, use it frequently. Take it at the same time every day to help with memory.

The dose is determined by your medical history, treatment response, and results of laboratory testing. For further information, speak with your doctor or pharmacist.

A variety of cyanocobalamin (vitamin B12) brands and dosage options are available. The quantity of cyanocobalamin (vitamin B12) in each product may vary, so read the dose guidelines thoroughly.

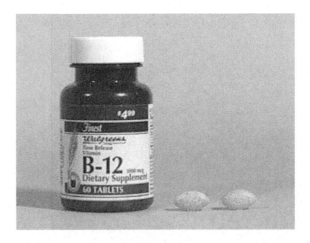

Use a specific measuring tool or spoon to precisely measure the dose if you are taking the drug in liquid form. Avoid using a regular spoon since you could not obtain the right dosage. You might need to thoroughly shake the container of certain liquid brands before each dose.

Do not chew or crush the extended-release pills while consuming them. This might cause the medicine to leak completely all at once, raising the possibility of negative effects.

Additionally, unless they have a score line and your doctor or pharmacist instructs you to do so, avoid splitting extended-release pills. Without crushing or chewing, take the full or divided pill.

If you're using a chewable tablet, make sure you chew it completely before swallowing.

If you're taking tablets that dissolve quickly, take them in your mouth with or without water as instructed by your physician or on the product label.

You may absorb fewer vitamin B12 if you consume vitamin C (ascorbic acid). Taking a lot of vitamin C an hour before or after taking this product is not advised.

Seek emergency medical assistance if your ailment persists or worsens, or if you suspect you may be suffering from a serious medical condition.

Side effects
In most cases, this product has no negative effects. Immediately get in touch with your doctor or pharmacist if you experience any odd symptoms.

If your doctor has prescribed this medicine for you, keep in mind that he or she has determined that the benefit to you outweighs the danger of adverse effects. Many users of this medicine report no significant negative effects.

As your body produces new red blood cells, this drug may occasionally result in low potassium levels in the blood (hypokalemia) if you have severe anemia. Muscle cramps, weakness, or an abnormal heartbeat are all uncommon but dangerous side effects that should be reported immediately to your doctor.

Rarely may this medication cause a very significant allergic response. However, if you have any signs of a major allergic response, such as a rash, itching or swelling (particularly of the face, tongue, or throat), severe dizziness, or difficulty breathing, you should seek emergency medical assistance.

The list of potential negative effects is not exhaustive. Contact your doctor or pharmacist if you have any other side effects not covered above.

Precautions
Inform your doctor or pharmacist if you have any allergies prior to taking cyanocobalamin, including those to cobalt, any form of vitamin B12, or any other type of vitamin.

Inactive chemicals in this product have the potential to trigger allergic reactions or other issues. To learn more, speak with your pharmacist.

Before using this drug, talk to your doctor or pharmacist if you have any of the following health issues: gout, iron- or folic-acid-deficiency anemia, Leber's visual neuropathy, polycythemia vera, a specific blood condition, and low potassium levels (hypokalemia).

Cyanocobalamin should only be administered orally if your body is capable of effectively absorbing it. If you suffer from pernicious anemia, issues with food absorption, stomach/intestinal surgery (such as gastric bypass or bowel resection), stomach/intestinal disease (such as Crohn's disease, colitis, diverticulitis, pancreatic insufficiency), or radiation to the small bowel, you may require a form of vitamin B12 that is injected or inhaled through the nose.

Inform your surgeon or dentist of all the products you use before surgery (including prescription drugs, nonprescription drugs, and herbal products).

When used at the prescribed dosages, cyanocobalamin is safe to use during pregnancy. Only take higher dosages if necessary. Describe the advantages and disadvantages to your doctor.

When administered in the prescribed doses, cyanocobalamin enters breast milk and is unlikely to damage a breastfeeding newborn. Before breastfeeding, speak with your doctor.

Interactions
If you use other medications or herbal remedies at the same time as some medications, the effects of those medications may alter. Your chance of experiencing major side effects

may arise as a result, and your medicine may also stop working as intended. Although certain medication interactions are conceivable, they don't usually happen. By modifying how you take your prescriptions or by closely monitoring you, your doctor or pharmacist can frequently avoid or manage interactions.

Before beginning therapy with this product, be sure to inform your doctor and pharmacist about all the items you use (including prescription medications, over-the-counter medicines, and herbal remedies). This will help them provide you with the best care possible. Do not begin, stop, or alter the dosage of any other medications you take while taking this product.

If you use other medications or herbal remedies at the same time as some medications, the effects of those medications may alter. Your chance of experiencing major side effects may arise as a result, and your medicine may also stop working as intended. Although certain medication interactions are conceivable, they don't usually happen. By modifying how you take your prescriptions or by closely monitoring you, your doctor or pharmacist can frequently avoid or manage interactions.

Before beginning therapy with this product, be sure to inform your doctor and pharmacist about all the items you use (including prescription medications, over-the-counter medicines, and herbal remedies). This will help them provide you with the best care possible. Do not begin, stop, or alter the dosage of any other medications you take while taking this product.

Drugs that impact the bone marrow, such as chloramphenicol, and vitamins and supplements that include intrinsic factors are a few examples of goods that may interact with this medication.

Colchicine, metformin, potassium products with extended-release, antibiotics (such as gentamicin, neomycin, and tobramycin), anti-seizure drugs (such as phenobarbital, phenytoin, and primidone), and medications for heartburn (such as H2 blockers like cimetidine/famotidine, proton pump inhibitors like omeprazole/lansoprazole) are just a few.

Many vitamin and dietary supplement products contain vitamin B12 as a component. If you're taking any other medications that include cyanocobalamin, vitamin B12, or hydroxocobalamin, let your doctor or pharmacist knows.

Cyanocobalamin may interfere with several laboratory tests (such as blood testing for intrinsic factor and other kinds of anemia), which might lead to inaccurate test findings. Make sure all of your physicians and the lab staff are aware that you use this medication.

Lab tests to measure vitamin B12 levels may be impacted by specific medicines, potentially leading to erroneous findings. If you take any of the following, inform the laboratory staff and all of your doctors: medicines (including erythromycin and amoxicillin), methotrexate, and pyrimethamine.

Conclusion

Pregnant women are more likely to have this deficit, especially if they are vegetarians. Constipation, breathlessness, and nausea are among the symptoms that frequently occur. The majority of individuals nowadays have succumbed to the fast food industry. Despite eating delectable cuisine, they are utterly deficient in the vitamins and minerals that the body needs to operate properly. Vegans are more likely to have vitamin B12 deficiencies than non-vegans since their diets lack adequate sources of this vitamin. Particularly young children and pregnant women are known to lack this essential nutrient for the body.

The extremely obvious and apparent symptoms include mouth sores, tingling or numbness in the limbs, palpitations, shortness of breath, nausea, and lack of appetite. Some people get mouth sores in addition to tingling on the tongue, which exacerbates the issue of appetite loss and ultimately results in weight loss. Due to his fatigue and extreme weakness, the person lacks interest in anything in life.

Additionally, sufferers may have fair skin. The primary transporters of oxygen to all the various cells and tissues of the body, red blood cells are the major culprits behind the development of these symptoms, according to medical professionals. Shortness of breath, palpitations, weakness, chest discomfort, etc. are all symptoms of an oxygen deficit in the body that results from decreased production of these cells.

This impairment has the potential to damage the gastrointestinal tract as well, which can cause a number of connected problems in the patients. Patients experience nausea, stomach bloating or enlargement, constipation, and other symptoms in acute situations. A lack of vitamin B12 damages the neural system as well, which results in symptoms including memory loss, tingling in the limbs, dementia, and depression.

Printed in Great Britain
by Amazon